ZOMBIE DEER DISEASE
UNMASKING THE SILENT MENACE

DECODING THE ENIGMA, UNDERSTANDING THE THREAT, AND CONFRONTING THE SHADOWS OF ZOMBIE DEER DISEASE

By

Daniel D. Belser

TABLE OF CONTENTS

INTRODUCTION

There is a menacing threat lurking in the quiet and shadowy American woodlands, giving the previously peaceful scenery an unsettling pallor. Some have dubbed it "Zombie Deer Disease," but the mystery illness has been silently spreading its tendrils and telling a terrifying story of ecological devastation that goes beyond the bounds of nature. We set out on a quest to solve the mystery of a silent scourge that has the power to fundamentally alter our perception of the natural world as we delve into the core of a growing wildlife crisis.

We uncover the layers of a biological mystery that calls into question our beliefs about the delicate ecosystems, the equilibrium between predator and prey, and the possible dangers that lurk just beyond our awareness as we explore the complexities of Chronic Wasting Disease (CWD), also known as Zombie Deer Disease. This book is a thorough examination into the causes, symptoms, and outcomes of a disease that affects the fundamental foundation of our natural environment, from the thick forests of the Pacific Northwest to the city centers of America.

Zombie Deer Disease is more than just a catchy name; it's a complicated network of biological relationships, research, and social ramifications. Through the history of epidemiology, public policy, and wildlife biology, we will explore the ramifications of CWD and learn about its riddles, which go much beyond the realm of animals.

We hope that our investigation will help us better comprehend the complexities of zombie deer disease and provide light on its larger significance for us as guardians of the fragile biodiversity of our world. The time has come to face the CWD specter and reveal the mysteries concealed in the eerie silence of the affected woodlands.

CHAPTER ONE

1.1 Purpose of the Book

We go into the particular objectives and motivations for writing this book about zombie deer disease in this section. The goal is to educate, enlighten, and increase awareness about the different aspects of CWD and its consequences for animal and human populations.

1. Knowledge Dissemination: The goal of this book is to provide readers—from members of the general public to experts in related fields—with a thorough grasp of Zombie Deer Disease by providing accurate and current information on the condition.

2. Public Awareness: By unraveling the complexities of CWD, the book attempts to promote public awareness about the possible risks connected with the condition, encouraging a sense of responsibility and urgency in tackling its issues.

3. Policy and Decision-Making: The book aims to assist policymakers in making well-informed decisions by offering

insights on the ethical, social, scientific, and economic aspects of zombie deer disease.

4. Research Catalyst: This book encourages continued attempts to expand our understanding of the condition and provide practical management solutions by acting as a spark for more study and investigation among scientists and researchers.

5. Mitigation Strategies: Upon completion, readers ought to possess a refined understanding of the illness, empowering them to take proactive steps towards prevention and make a positive impact on the general reduction of Zombie Deer Disease.

1.2 Scope and Limitations:

To control expectations and appreciate the breadth of coverage on Zombie Deer Disease, readers must be aware of the scope and limitations of this book.

Range:

1. Scientific Exploration: This book delves deeply into the scientific elements of Zombie Deer Disease, offering a comprehensive analysis of the disease's genesis, dynamics of transmission, and distinctive features associated with prion illnesses.

2. Implications for Human Health: The scope includes a thorough examination of the possible effects of Zombie Deer Disease on human health, taking into account verified case reports, transmission pathways, and zoonotic potential.

3. Interdisciplinary Approach: Giving a comprehensive view of the complex nature of CWD, the book explores issues beyond the scientific domain, such as public awareness, government actions, socioeconomic ramifications, and ethical issues.

4. Preventive Measures: Readers will discover useful information on safety procedures for hunters, best practices for managing venison, and suggestions for scientists and veterinarians working on the disease's research or treatment.

Restrictions:

1. Evolution of Knowledge: As new discoveries are made, some of the knowledge contained in this book may become out of date due to the dynamic nature of scientific study. It is recommended that readers keep up with the most recent advancements in the subject.

2. Geographical Focus: Although attempts are undertaken to discuss the worldwide ramifications of zombie deer disease, the book might primarily concentrate on areas where the illness is more common. The currently available data restricts consideration of its impact in other geographical locations.

3. Thorough Policy Coverage: Although the book offers insights into official reactions and rules, it might not address all policy nuances or regional variations pertaining to zombie deer disease. It is recommended that readers examine individual policy documents for more comprehensive details.

4. Ethical Issues: Although ethical issues are included in the book, it might not address all ethical problems related to zombie deer disease. The dynamic nature of ethical discourse may give rise to further ideas that go outside the book's purview.

This book seeks to provide readers with a realistic expectation of its material while encouraging a critical approach to studying Zombie Deer Disease by outlining its extent and identifying its limitations.

CHAPTER TWO

2.1 Origin and Discovery of Zombie Deer Disease

The disease formerly known as Chronic Wasting Disease (CWD), or zombie deer disease, was first identified and discovered in the late 20th century, mostly in the western regions of the United States. The disease was initially identified in the 1960s in captive mule deer at a Colorado research facility; nevertheless, it was not until the 1980s that researchers and wildlife management acknowledged it as a unique and concerning phenomenon. The disease caused deer to exhibit puzzling symptoms at first, such as emaciation, drowsiness, and a distinctive drooping of the ears. After a thorough analysis of these peculiar symptoms, scientists were able to differentiate CWD from other wildlife diseases by identifying prions—a manifold protein—as the causal culprit.

Scientists like Drs. Elizabeth Williams and Richard Race, who conducted groundbreaking research, were instrumental in characterizing Zombie Deer Disease. Early on in the disease's discovery, scientists had trouble comprehending how it spread and how it would affect wildlife populations. An important advancement was the creation of specialized methods, such as the use of transgenic mice to investigate prion 'infectivity'. In the years that followed, more study was conducted, which helped to clarify the geographic distribution of CWD and its effects on other cervid species, such as elk and deer. This groundbreaking era in the study of zombie deer sickness laid the groundwork for a more comprehensive comprehension of prion diseases and their effects on animal and human health.

The development of knowledge on Zombie Deer Disease highlighted the multidisciplinary character of research in the domains of neurology, veterinary medicine, and wildlife biology. The discovery of CWD spurred increasing cooperation between government agencies, academic institutions, and wildlife management organizations as scientists wrestled with the particular issues provided by prion diseases. The early findings that impacted our knowledge of the origins and complexities of Zombie Deer Disease continue to inform continuing efforts to monitor and control the disease.

2.2 Causes and Transmission of Zombie Deer Disease

Prion diseases, also referred to as chronic wasting disease (CWD) in science, are the cause of zombie deer disease. Prions are manifold proteins that, in contrast to more common infectious agents like bacteria or viruses, can cause their host's normal cellular proteins to misfold as well. These prions primarily impact the central nervous system in the case of CWD, resulting in neurodegeneration and the typical symptoms seen in infected deer, including emaciation, aberrant behavior, and a vacant gaze. Science is still investigating the genesis of prions in the environment, their persistence, and the mechanisms that cause them to change from normal to pathological states.

There are two ways that Zombie Deer Disease spreads: directly and indirectly. Close contact between an infected and an uninfected person can result in the exchange of bodily fluids, including urine, feces, and saliva. This is known as direct transmission. This can happen in social situations, during mating, or when contaminated settings are shared. Prions can remain infectious in the environment for a long time, which makes indirect transmission easier. Deer that eat infected plants, soil, or water sources may be exposed to CWD prions. Concerns concerning the long-term dangers connected to regions where diseased deer have been present are raised by prions' capacity to endure in the environment.

Creating efficient management and prevention plans requires an understanding of the intricate dynamics of CWD transmission. The management of deer populations, the implementation of surveillance systems, the establishment of regulations for hunters, and the handling of games are all part of the efforts to slow the spread of zombie deer disease. A more all-encompassing strategy for managing this difficult illness is emerging as further study expands our understanding of the causes and dynamics of transmission while balancing ecological preservation with public health concerns.

2.3 Signs and Symptoms in Deer

Within afflicted deer populations, the symptoms of Zombie Deer Disease, formerly known as Chronic Wasting Disease (CWD), present in different ways. Unnoticed in the early stages of illness, observable indications grow more prominent as the disease advances. Emaciation or the loss of weight gradually and severely, is one of the main signs. A lack of coordination, a marked disinterest in their environment, and repetitive walking in predetermined patterns are examples of odd behaviors seen by infected deer. Affected deer frequently exhibit excessive salivation, drooping ears, and a vacant, glassy-eyed stare as the disease progresses, adding to the unsettling picture that led to the disease's unofficial moniker, "Zombie Deer Disease."

Infected deer often suffer from neurological problems, such as a breakdown in normal brain function that impairs their ability to react appropriately to stimuli. As a result, these animals might no longer be afraid of people and exhibit changed social behaviors, underscoring the terrible effects of CWD on the animals' general health. The complicated ecological effects of

Zombie Deer Disease in wildlife populations are exacerbated when these symptoms worsen and make afflicted deer more susceptible to predators and environmental stressors.

2.4 Spread and Geography of Zombie Deer Disease

The spread of Chronic Wasting Disease (CWD), also known as Zombie Deer Disease (ZDDD), has become a serious public health and wildlife management issue. When the disease was first discovered, it was only found in a small region of the country, mostly in the West. However, it has shown a concerning ability to spread over time. As of right now, reports of CWD have been made in cervid populations in the wild and in captivity throughout North America, including parts of Canada and Mexico. The adaptability and tenacity of CWD present serious obstacles for authorities trying to stop its spread and lessen its effects on ecosystems.

Vigilant surveillance and monitoring are required because of the dynamic and ever-evolving geographical distribution of CWD. Prions can be released into the environment by infected deer through their body fluids, which can contaminate the surrounding plants and soil. This environmental persistence presents a special difficulty since CWD can spread to new places through the movement of sick deer or human activities like the transportation of contaminated carcasses. It can also remain infectious for years. It is more difficult to anticipate and manage the regional spread of zombie deer disease because of the intricate interactions between environmental conditions, population dynamics, and human activity.

Comprehending the transmission of CWD is essential for evaluating possible hazards to human populations as well as for the preservation of wildlife. The disease's capacity to transcend species boundaries and its documented existence in areas where hunters and outdoor enthusiasts frequently highlight the significance of all-encompassing approaches to control and lessen the disease's geographic impact. Working together at the local, national, and international levels is crucial to addressing the complex issues brought about by the rising geographic scope of this worrying wildlife disease.

CHAPTER THREE

The Science Behind Zombie Deer Disease

The complex field of prion biology is at the center of the research on Zombie Deer Disease (CWD), also known by its scientific name. The erroneous folding of typical cellular proteins—most notably the prion protein (PrP)—into aberrant, infectious forms is the fundamental cause of this disease. The strange property of these manifold proteins, known as prions, is that they may cause other healthy proteins to wrongly fold as well, starting a domino effect that leads to the buildup of aberrant protein aggregates in the brain. In the case of CWD, these prions wreak havoc on the central nervous system of deer, leading to 'neurodegeneration' and the specific symptoms noticed in infected people. The transmission of prions, their environmental persistence, and the intricate interactions between genetic and environmental factors that impact disease susceptibility and development are all explored in the study of CWD.

In order to fully understand the complexity of this prion-based disease, researchers studying Zombie Deer Disease use a multidisciplinary approach that combines molecular biology, genetics, epidemiology, and ecology. The discovery of CWD prions in body fluids including urine and saliva highlights the possibility of deer-to-deer direct transmission.

Furthermore, a special problem is presented by the environmental persistence of prions, since contaminated soil and plants serve as harbors for infectious particles. Current scientific efforts are directed at improving diagnostic instruments, comprehending the variables affecting the geographical dissemination of CWD, and investigating possible treatment approaches. The scientific study of Zombie Deer Disease highlights the wider consequences for ecosystems, public health, and animals in addition to providing insight into the mechanisms underlying this mysterious illness.

3.1 Prion Diseases Explained

A distinct family of neurodegenerative illnesses known as prions diseases is defined by the aberrant, infectious folding of normal cellular proteins. Prion infectious pathogens lack genetic material, in contrast to more common infectious agents like bacteria or viruses. In fact, the word "prion" itself comes from the word "proteinaceous infectious particle." The cellular protein PrP (prion protein), which makes up the majority of the manifold prion proteins, catalyzes the erroneous folding of normal PrP proteins, which sets off a chain reaction that results in the buildup of aberrant protein aggregates in the brain. The normal cellular function is disrupted by this accumulation, leading to gradual and irreversible damage to neuronal tissues.

Prions are transmissible within and between species, which is one of their unique characteristics. Through direct contact between people, eating infected tissues, or being in places where prions are present, the infectious prion particles can spread. Many animals, including humans, are susceptible to prion illnesses, which have distinct symptoms for each species. Apart from Zombie Deer Disease (also known as Chronic Wasting Disease), other notable cases are Creutzfeldt-Jakob Disease (CJD) in humans and Bovine Spongiform Encephalopathy (BSE, also known as "mad cow disease") in cattle. The intricate interactions between genetic, environmental, and molecular factors are responsible for the various ways that prion diseases present themselves in different species.

The transformation of normal, soluble PrP proteins into insoluble, aggregated forms is the basic underpinning of prion disorders. The result of this conversion is the development of characteristic microscopic formations known as amyloid plaques, which are indicative of prion pathology. Even while prion diseases appear to have a straightforward constitution, their distinct routes of transmission, subtle development, and lack of typical immune responses pose complex hurdles for researchers and physicians. Current research endeavors are focused on deciphering the intricacies of prion disorders, augmenting our comprehension of their biology, and opening the door for possible remedial measures.

3.2 Unique Characteristics of Zombie Deer Prions

The infectious organisms that cause Chronic Wasting Disease (CWD), known as zombie deer prions, differ from traditional pathogens in a number of ways. Prions have no genetic material; instead, they are made entirely of manifold proteins, unlike bacteria or viruses. The remarkable resistance of zombie deer prions to conventional cleaning techniques is what sets them apart from other prions. These prions are difficult to eradicate because they can withstand extreme environmental factors like heat and chemical treatments. Their tenacity in the environment is facilitated by this resilience, which also presents a sustained danger of transmission to deer and maybe other animals.

The capacity of zombie deer prions to transcend interspecies boundaries is another distinctive feature. Although cervids, such as deer and elk, are the primary victims of CWD, experimental research has shown that, in some situations, other mammals may also contract the disease. Worries concerning the wider ramifications for human health are raised by this zoonotic potential. It is essential to comprehend the unique characteristics of zombie deer prions in order to create management plans and preventative measures that work. In order to reduce the risk to human populations and lessen the impact of CWD on wildlife, ongoing research aims to understand the molecular details that give rise to these prions' resistance, transmissibility, and ability to adapt to various host species.

3.3 Research and Studies of Zombie Deer Disease

The scientific community has increased the number of research routes and studies it has conducted in an attempt to better comprehend zombie deer disease. Studies have been conducted to investigate prospective treatment strategies, transmission patterns, and the molecular details of prion proteins linked to Chronic Wasting Disease (CWD). Researchers are able to analyze the intricate processes that underlie the onset, spread, and pathophysiology of CWD thanks to technological advancements in laboratory procedures such as sophisticated imaging technology and molecular biology tools.

In order to map the spread of zombie deer disease and evaluate its effects on wildlife populations, epidemiological studies are essential. To determine susceptible populations, track the geographic distribution of CWD, and comprehend the variables affecting disease occurrence, researchers utilize genetic analyses, field studies, and monitoring systems. Studies on the zoonotic potential of CWD are being conducted concurrently in an effort to assess the dangers to human health. In order to improve our knowledge of CWD and develop evidence-based methods for disease management and prevention, scientists, wildlife biologists, veterinarians, and public health specialists collaborate on these research projects. Ongoing study offers insightful information that could aid in the creation of practical solutions to lessen the effects of zombie deer disease on both wildlife and human populations.

CHAPTER FOUR

The Potential Impact on Human Health

Research on the possible effects of Chronic Wasting Disease (CWD), also known as Zombie Deer Disease (ZDD), on human health is ongoing and is becoming increasingly of great concern. Although definitive proof of direct CWD transmission to humans is still lacking, prion diseases, of which CWD is a member, have the potential to spread to humans, which has led to the implementation of preventive measures. Cross-species transmission is possible because studies have demonstrated that the CWD-causing prions can adapt to new species in an experimental setting. As a result, people who could be more vulnerable to exposure—such as hunters and people who eat meat from diseased deer—are being watched more closely. In order to evaluate the risk and comprehend any possible consequences for public health, monitoring and surveillance activities are essential. The possible effects of CWD on human health are still being studied, but they highlight the necessity of taking preventative steps to reduce exposure, guarantee the security of food sources, and keep an eye on communities that are at risk.

4.1 Zoonotic potential

Chronic Wasting Disease (CWD), the former name of Zombie Deer Disease (ZD), has drawn intense scientific attention and public health scrutiny due to its possible zoonotic threat. Despite the lack of conclusive data at this time supporting CWD transmission to humans, the distinct features of prion diseases, of which CWD is one, raise questions regarding the possibility of cross-species transmission. The ability of CWD prions to adapt to new species has been shown in laboratory trials, which raises the prospect of zoonotic transmission in some situations. Due to this, people who have had direct contact with infected animals—especially hunters and others who eat venison from deer populations in places where CWD is common—are being closely watched.

Numerous investigations, including genetic analysis, epidemiological research, and population surveillance of humans and wildlife, are being conducted to evaluate the zoonotic potential of Zombie Deer Disease. Public health guidelines are based on the precautionary principle, which emphasizes the significance of reducing exposure to potentially hazardous sources. To lower any possible dangers, regulatory bodies, and health authorities give hunters and venison processors guidance. The dynamic nature of scientific knowledge emphasizes the necessity of ongoing investigations to thoroughly evaluate the zoonotic potential of CWD, guaranteeing a proactive and knowledgeable strategy to protect human health.

4.2 Mechanisms of Transmission of Zombie Deer Disease to Humans

Research on the processes of Chronic Wasting Disease (CWD), sometimes known as zombie deer disease, and its transmission to humans is an intricate and dynamic field. As prion diseases have the potential to spread to humans, CWD is one of those diseases. However, the precise processes by which the disease could do so remain to be completely understood.

Direct Transmission Pathways:

The main area of worry is the possibility of direct infection spreading from infected deer to humans. There may be a risk if humans come into contact with bodily fluids from infected animals, such as blood, urine, or saliva. Hunters, wildlife experts, and people engaged in deer farming are especially at risk of exposure as they have frequent contact with diseased animals. There is still research being done to determine how much of the prions found in these body fluids can infect people and pass the species barrier.

2. Consumption of Contaminated Meat: Another way that humans may contract the disease is by eating venison from diseased deer. The brain, spinal cord, lymph nodes, and muscles of sick deer are among the specific regions where prions linked to chronic deer weakness (CWD) might collect. Cooking helps lower infection risk, but it doesn't completely get rid of prions. Because of this, hunting instructions frequently advise against eating specific tissues, especially those with greater prion concentrations, in order to reduce potential dangers.

3. Environmental Contamination: The transmission dynamics are further complicated by the environmental persistence of CWD prions. Humans may be indirectly in danger from contaminated soil, water sources, and vegetation in places that infected deer frequently visit. Research is still being done on the possibility that people could come into touch with these environmental reservoirs and then contract the infection.

4. Zoonotic Adaptation: The capacity of prions to adapt to novel species affects the zoonotic potential of CWD. The ability of CWD prions to adapt has been shown in experimental research, which raises questions regarding the potential for cross-species transmission. Research is still being done on the circumstances behind this adaptation and the possibility of long-term transfer to humans.

4.3 Case Studies and Incidents of Zombie Deer Disease in Humans

According to the most recent data available, there have been no reported cases of Chronic Wasting Disease (CWD), sometimes known as zombie deer disease, in people. Cervids, such as deer and elk, are the primary victims of CWD, and studies and monitoring are ongoing to determine how the disease can spread to humans. It is crucial to remember, though, that prion diseases—of which CWD is one—have shown the ability to spread from animals to humans in specific situations.

The comparatively lengthy incubation periods linked to prion disorders and the paucity of comprehensive data on human exposure provide significant obstacles to research on the zoonotic potential of CWD. Even after much investigation, there is still no solid proof that CWD and human prion illnesses like Creutzfeldt-Jakob Disease (CJD) are related.

A number of case studies and occurrences have examined people who may have come into contact with animals infected with CWD. Research has, for instance, concentrated on hunters who frequently eat venison from deer populations in areas where chronic wasting disease is common. The purpose of these studies is to monitor the health of those who are more likely to be exposed and to evaluate any possible abnormalities connected to prion disease or the nervous system. Even though no examples of CWD transmission to humans have been found as a result of these studies, the research highlights the significance of continuous surveillance and the requirement for preventive actions to reduce potential dangers.

It is critical to evaluate case studies in light of the larger framework of our developing knowledge of prion biology and zombie deer disease. Public health policies will continue to depend on tracking human populations at risk of CWD exposure and improving preventive measures. Researchers and public health organizations work together to develop hunting rules, distribute information about safe consumption techniques, and carry out in-depth inquiries into any events that can give rise to worries about the human-to-duck transmission of CWD.

CHAPTER FIVE

Government Response and Regulations

Governments at the local, state, and federal levels have responded to the alarming rise in chronic wasting disease (CWD), also known as "zombie deer disease," by enacting various regulations and measures aimed at stopping the disease's spread. CWD is a neurodegenerative sickness that affects deer, elk, and moose. Authorities have launched extensive monitoring operations to track and identify affected animals because they are aware of the possible negative effects on the environment and the economy. To reduce human-assisted transmission, strict hunting laws and carcass disposal procedures have also been implemented. In order to create efficient management plans, governments are working with academic institutions to expand their knowledge of the biology and dynamics of the disease's transmission. In order to inform communities about the dangers of CWD and the need to follow suggested recommendations, more intense public awareness campaigns and outreach programs are being implemented. Governments are diligent in adjusting their actions to address the effects of zombie deer disease on wildlife populations and protect public health, even as the scientific community continues to explore the disease.

5.1 Surveillance and Monitoring

The scientific term for zombie deer sickness is chronic wasting disease (CWD), and government initiatives to stop its spread and comprehend its dynamics currently heavily rely on surveillance and monitoring activities. Comprehensive surveillance systems that include systematic testing of moose, elk, and deer populations have been created throughout the impacted regions. This includes roadkill specimen monitoring, testing requirements for harvested animals, and targeted sampling during hunting seasons. Authorities can quickly identify and address new cases by prioritizing and identifying high-risk regions for increased surveillance. Modern technologies are used to improve the precision and effectiveness of CWD identification, including genetic testing and sophisticated diagnostics. Systems for collecting and analyzing data in real-time make it easier to identify diseased animals quickly, which helps to apply targeted management measures. The sharing of surveillance data across federal, state, and local organizations promotes cooperation in the fight against the illness.

Additionally, research is being done to identify locations with a higher risk of CWD transmission through the development of non-invasive monitoring techniques including soil and vegetation analysis. Refinement and expansion of monitoring systems are priorities for governments as surveillance plays a critical role in combating zombie deer disease. This will enable them to respond to the danger to wildlife health in a proactive and flexible manner.

5.2 Emergency Measures

Governments have implemented emergency protocols to handle chronic wasting disease (CWD), often known as zombie deer illness, in an effort to control and lessen the effects of this wildlife health emergency. Upon confirmation of cases, prompt containment measures are initiated, which frequently entail creating restricted areas and imposing mobility restrictions on cervid populations in both captivity and the wild. In severely impacted areas, depopulation techniques may be used, including the culling of diseased and vulnerable animals to stop the spread of the illness. To quickly and effectively coordinate these activities, emergency response teams made up of veterinarians, law enforcement, and specialists in wildlife conservation are called in.

Public outreach and education initiatives are launched in tandem with containment measures to educate the public about the dangers of CWD and to promote adherence to preventive measures. Guidelines for the appropriate handling and disposal of corpses are often included in emergency response plans, with an emphasis on the necessity of reducing the amount of transmission that occurs with human assistance. One of the main components of these emergency measures is the establishment of stringent hunting laws, which include heightened surveillance throughout hunting seasons. Governments work in tandem with academic institutions and veterinary specialists to continuously evaluate the changing circumstances and modify emergency protocols as necessary to protect public health and wildlife populations.

5.3 Policy Development

Policy creation in response to zombie deer disease, or chronic wasting disease (CWD), has become a priority for governments attempting to construct comprehensive and effective frameworks to fight this animal health concern. These regulations usually take a multifaceted approach, including management, preventative, and surveillance techniques. Authorities collaborate closely with stakeholders, epidemiologists, and wildlife specialists to develop evidence-based policies that specifically address the problems caused by CWD. These policies frequently involve steps to improve surveillance, make use of cutting-edge technologies for early diagnosis, and set up procedures for the correct management and disposal of diseased animals. In order to reduce the risk of disease spread, regulatory frameworks are also put in place to regulate the movement of moose, elk, and deer populations. These frameworks include tight requirements for handling carcasses and transporting live animals.

Public awareness campaigns, in which governments actively participate in teaching communities about the dangers of CWD and the significance of adhering to established norms, are another aspect of policy creation. These regulations might provide rewards to hunters who provide samples for analysis, encouraging openness and collaboration between public authorities and the general people. Policy evolution depends on ongoing research collaboration with scientific institutions to ensure that laws remain flexible in response to the changing nature of zombie deer disease. Governments hope to establish a holistic policy framework that efficiently manages chronic wasting disease (CWD), preserves wildlife populations, and protects public health by incorporating these disparate elements.

CHAPTER SIX

Social and Economic Implications

Chronic wasting disease (CWD), also referred to as zombie deer illness, has broad and profound social and economic effects. Socially, the disease presents problems for nearby populations that depend on wildlife- and hunting-related activities since it may result in fewer opportunities for cervid hunting and other cervid-related recreational activities. In addition to raising concerns about public health and safety, the possibility of CWD transmission to people calls for increased awareness and protective measures. Budgets for wildlife management may be impacted financially by the disease because of the need for more testing, surveillance, and response work.

Additionally, companies that depend on hunting and wildlife viewing could be impacted by the possible reduction in cervid populations, which would have a knock-on effect on the local economy. The wider ramifications highlight the necessity of a comprehensive strategy to lessen the social and financial effects of zombie deer illness, striking a balance between efficient disease control and the protection of livelihoods and public health.

6.1 Perception and Public Awareness

Chronic Wasting sickness (CWD), the formal name for zombie deer sickness, has drawn a lot of attention from the public and sparked worries about its possible effects on wildlife and public health. As CWD cases keep popping up in different parts of the country, people's knowledge about this illness has significantly increased. Information regarding the nature of CWD, how it spreads, and any possible risks have been widely disseminated by government agencies, wildlife organizations, and health authorities to the general public.

The general public's opinions and perceptions of zombie deer illness vary widely, despite these attempts. Because the disease causes the nervous system of infected deer to deteriorate, some people experience increased anxiety and terror and compare it to a situation similar to that of a zombie. Some people could minimize the seriousness of the problem, seeing it as a confined issue with only minor effects on human health. Finding the right balance between disseminating correct information and preventing unwarranted alarms is still difficult. To promote responsible wildlife management practices and informed decision-making, it is imperative to cultivate a shared awareness of the disease, its causes, and the actions implemented to curb its spread.

6.2 Economic Impact on Local Communities

Beyond the immediate concerns for wildlife health, zombie deer illness, also known as Chronic Wasting illness (CWD), has a complex economic impact on nearby populations. Due to CWD's effects on deer populations and the resulting limits on hunting in afflicted areas, one of the main economic ramifications is the possible loss in hunting-related revenue. Businesses that serve hunters, such as outfitters, motels, restaurants, and other establishments, may see a decline in business during a downturn in local economies that strongly depend on hunting tourism and related industries. Additionally, the stigma attached to CWD may discourage travelers and outdoor enthusiasts, which would hurt the local tourism industry as a whole.

Apart from the immediate impact on the outdoor recreation sector, there exist secondary economic ramifications associated with wildlife conservation initiatives and agricultural matters. The state and local governments must spend more money on containment measures and monitoring programs, which takes funds away from other community initiatives. Additionally,

CWD may have an effect on livestock husbandry due to the possibility of stricter regulations and more inspection due to worries about disease transfer from deer to domestic animals. The economic effects of zombie deer sickness underscore the interdependence of the local economy, animal health, and the careful balancing act necessary to appropriately handle these scenarios.

6.3 Challenges in Livestock Management

The advent and dissemination of Chronic Wasting illness (CWD), often known as zombie deer illness, presents significant obstacles in the field of animal management. The possible spread of CWD prions from diseased deer to domesticated animals is one of the main worries. cattle farmers are left in a state of uncertainty as the scientific community is actively investigating the possible risk despite the lack of conclusive evidence of direct transmission to cattle. Due to customer worries about food safety, producers may find it difficult to market their products, which could have an impact on the economy.

The testing and regulatory requirements for animals are just one aspect of the complex management of CWD. Stricter regulations may be implemented by governments and agricultural organizations to track and manage the disease's spread. Livestock farmers may find their resources stretched by more testing and surveillance, which could result in higher operating expenses and possible disruptions to regular farming procedures. Furthermore, it becomes imperative to implement strong 'biosecurity' protocols to avoid unintentionally exposing tamed animals to regions where diseased deer could have previously resided. The issues in livestock management owing to zombie deer illness show the complicated relationship between wildlife health and domestic agriculture, and the need for a multidisciplinary approach to handle the possible risks and repercussions for the livestock business.

CHAPTER SEVEN

Humanitarian and Ethical Considerations

The scientific term for zombie deer disease is Chronic Wasting Disease (CWD), and it raises severe ethical and humanitarian problems about how human safety, wildlife health, and moral wildlife management practices all intersect. Amidst the mystery surrounding the transfer of prions that cause CWD, concerns regarding possible health hazards to humans emerge as the disease's effects persist on deer populations. Addressing the disease's spread raises ethical questions since control techniques like reducing diseased deer herds can spark discussions about how humanely to treat wildlife. It is a difficult task to strike a balance between the need to preserve wildlife and human health while upholding moral principles. This calls for a methodical and well-informed strategy that takes into account the well-being of both people and the impacted animal species.

7.1 Dealing with Stigma and Fear

It is imperative to tackle the fear and stigma associated with Chronic Wasting Disease (CWD), sometimes known as zombie deer disease, in order to promote a knowledgeable public opinion and execute efficient management tactics. Misconceptions regarding the human-to-deer transmission of CWD and the overly dramatic association of afflicted deer with a "zombie-like" condition are frequent causes of public fear. In order to debunk misconceptions and provide factual information about the illness, public health organizations and wildlife advocacy groups are essential. Cooperation in disseminating the scientific understanding of CWD, with a focus on the fact that there isn't any proof of transfer to humans yet, can help allay unfounded anxieties and lessen the stigma associated with damaged wildlife.

Initiatives for education and community involvement are also crucial in tackling stigma and fear. Giving communities clear and easy access to information on CWD, its causes, and current management initiatives can encourage them to take an active role in both disease prevention and wildlife conservation. Public discourse can become more sophisticated by supporting a balanced narrative about the condition and encouraging media sources to report responsibly. In order to promote a more accurate image of zombie deer sickness and facilitate collaborative efforts for its effective management, stakeholders can collaborate to lessen the effects of fear and stigma around the disease by creating an environment that values understanding and cooperation.

7.2 Ethical Treatment of Infected Wildlife

For wildlife management authorities, the moral treatment of afflicted wildlife in the context of chronic wasting disease (CWD), often known as zombie deer illness, presents a difficult problem. When creating ethical rules for handling diseased animals, it is important to strike a balance between the necessity of disease management and humane concerns. In regions where CWD is highly prevalent, depopulation techniques like culling are frequently used to stop the disease from spreading; however, there are moral questions about how these animals should be handled humanely. Governments work to reduce suffering as much as possible. For example, they use sharpshooters to guarantee prompt and effective culling and use veterinary knowledge to improve depopulation tactics. Furthermore, when disposing of carcasses, ethical considerations must be taken into account. Scavengers must be kept away from contaminated remains in order to minimize environmental contamination.

Research exploring alternate strategies, such as the creation of vaccinations or therapies to control the disease within wild populations without resorting to mass culling, is becoming more and more important in the ethical treatment of affected species.

This strategy complies with moral precepts that put animal welfare first, even when disease control is involved. It is a constant struggle to strike a balance between managing the disease and providing ethical care. To this end, veterinarians, ethicists, and wildlife experts must work together to develop strategies that not only effectively reduce CWD but also uphold the values of compassion and respect for wildlife.

7.3 Balancing Conservation and Public Health

In the context of zombie deer disease, also known as chronic wasting disease (CWD), striking a balance between public health concerns and conservation is a complex problem. On the one hand, strong conservation efforts are desperately needed to protect cervid populations and the environments they live in. Proactive steps are needed to stop the illness from spreading outside of wildlife, though, as the possibility of CWD spreading to people poses serious public health issues. Wildlife management authorities must put procedures into place that both minimize the risk of human exposure and lessen the impact of CWD on cervid populations in order to strike the correct balance. This could entail developing adaptive management strategies, combining intensive surveillance with targeted culling in high-risk areas, and creating preventive measures that take into account the issue's ecological and public health implications.

Finding this equilibrium is greatly aided by effective communication, which raises public awareness of the intricacies involved. Transparent communication is employed by governments and health organizations to inform populations about the science underlying CWD, the dynamics of its transmission, and the importance of certain conservation actions. A comprehensive strategy that tackles the competing demands of public health and conservation is further enhanced by cooperative research projects involving wildlife specialists and public health specialists. Authorities can work toward sustainable solutions that safeguard human populations as well as wildlife environments by navigating the complex interactions between these factors.

CHAPTER EIGHT

Preventive Measures and Safety Protocols

Comprehensive methods designed to reduce the risk of disease transmission to humans and wildlife must include preventive measures and safety practices for chronic wasting disease (CWD), often known as zombie deer sickness. With an emphasis on reducing the transmission of the disease with human assistance, authorities enforce stringent regulations governing the handling and shipping of cervid species. Testing of harvested animals is required as part of safety procedures during hunting and processing, and carcass disposal rules are in place to protect the environment from contamination. Campaigns for public awareness stress the need to report sick or unusual-looking animals and forbid eating meat from cervids that are afflicted. In addition, research is being conducted to investigate alternate preventive methods that target the underlying cause of CWD in addition to developing vaccines and therapies for the disease. The joint endeavors of wildlife management agencies, public health organizations, and communities facilitate the development and execution of safety protocols and preventive measures that are intended to protect animal populations and public health.

8.1 Recommendations for Hunters

In the context of chronic wasting disease (CWD), often known as zombie deer disease, hunting recommendations are essential for stopping the disease's spread and protecting the health of the population and wildlife alike. First and foremost, hunters are urged to report any animals displaying strange behavior or symptoms suggestive of CWD and to remain alert. It is highly recommended that harvested animals take part in voluntary testing programs, as this aids wildlife management authorities in tracking the disease's incidence and taking appropriate action to stop its spread. Hunters should also observe local laws on the transportation and disposal of carcasses, making sure that the right procedures are followed to reduce the possibility of infectious prions, which cause CWD, spreading.

Second, it is recommended that hunters handle the game they have harvested in a responsible and safe manner. Because CWD can spread to humans, this includes avoiding eating meat from animals that seem ill or odd. It is advised to take safety precautions such as thoroughly cleaning and disinfecting processing-related equipment and limiting contact with brain and spinal tissues, which have a greater concentration of infectious prions. The dissemination of these suggestions is greatly aided by public awareness efforts, which highlight the shared duty of hunters in halting the spread of zombie deer illness while protecting the integrity of wildlife populations and public health.

8.2 Guidelines for Handling Venison

To reduce the possibility of transmission to humans, guidelines for managing venison in the context of chronic wasting disease (CWD), also known as zombie deer disease, are essential. Authorities advise hunters to proceed with caution when field dressing, being careful not to come into contact with high-risk tissues including the spinal cord and brain, which are known to contain infectious prions. In order to avoid cross-contamination, hunters should also completely clean and sanitize knives, cutting surfaces, and other processing equipment. Cutting through bones can increase the risk of prion exposure, hence it is recommended to bone out the flesh from harvested animals instead of sawing through them. It's important to note that before eating the venison, hunters are urged to have their harvested animals tested for CWD. It is advised to completely refrain from eating the meat if an animal tests positive.

Guidelines also emphasize the significance of using appropriate cooking and storage techniques. In order to prevent infection, hunters should handle food safely and store venison apart from other animal flesh. It is highly advised to cook venison all the way through to an internal temperature of at least 160°F (71°C), as heat has the power to eradicate the prions that cause chronic wasting disease. These thorough guidelines support a responsible and knowledgeable approach to controlling the hazards connected with zombie deer illness by highlighting the dual goals of enjoying venison while guaranteeing the safety of individuals who consume it.

8.3 Protective Measures for Researchers and Veterinarians

To maintain the integrity of research projects and the safety of scientists and veterinarians studying chronic wasting disease (CWD), or zombie deer illness, protective measures are essential. When handling cervid specimens or doing post-mortem investigations, researchers and veterinarians are required to use gloves, masks, and protective clothes as a first line of defense known as personal protective equipment (PPE). This lowers the chance of skin and mucous membrane contamination as well as the risk of direct contact with potentially infectious objects.

Using biosafety-level-rated laboratories with specific ventilation systems reduces the possibility of CWD spreading through the air in laboratory settings. In order to prevent cross-contamination, decontamination standards for tools, surfaces, and work areas are strictly adhered to. Additionally, researchers receive comprehensive training on identifying symptoms of CWD and putting appropriate handling measures in place to reduce exposure risks.

Protective measures also include continual education and risk management in addition to physical precautions. In order to stay up to date on the most recent advancements in the area, researchers and veterinarians working on CWD studies undergo ongoing training. They also acquire techniques for handling unintentional exposures or possible infections. Health monitoring is regularly carried out to detect and swiftly address any developing hazards, including routine testing for exposure to CWD. The psychological health of researchers investigating CWD is also taken into account, and resources such as counseling and support services are made available to help with the particular difficulties that come with researching a disease that has complicated ethical and scientific aspects.

Protective measures for researchers and veterinarians on zombie deer disease not only improve the safety of those involved but also contribute to the overall success and dependability of CWD research efforts through a combination of strict safety protocols, ongoing training, and a holistic approach to well-being.

CONCLUSION

CALL TO ACTION

Zombie deer disease, also known as chronic wasting disease (CWD), is a condition that requires immediate attention and coordinated action since it crosses the boundaries between public health and wildlife conservation. Given that CWD is becoming more common in deer populations in different countries, it is critical to coordinate efforts to address the many issues this transmissible neurological illness presents. In order to combat the threat of CWD and protect human and wildlife populations, stakeholders—including government agencies, wildlife organizations, researchers, and the general public—can take the important actions outlined in this call to action.

1. Increase Public Awareness and Education: Providing the public with accurate and easily accessible information is a crucial first step in reducing the effects of CWD. Together, government departments and animal advocacy groups

should launch extensive public education campaigns that debunk misconceptions, explain the true dangers of CWD, and advocate for ethical wildlife management. Communities will become more knowledgeable and able to actively participate in disease prevention and monitoring initiatives if they are educated about the disease, its routes of transmission, and preventative measures.

2. Invest in Research and Monitoring: More money must be spent on research in order to effectively combat CWD. This entails funding research on the mechanics of the disease's spread, creating trustworthy diagnostic instruments, and investigating cutting-edge management techniques that put the welfare of animal populations and moral treatment first. Establishing robust monitoring programs will help track the spread of CWD and enable early discovery and quick action. Evidence-based management strategies will be informed by collaborative research projects including wildlife biologists, veterinarians, and public health specialists, leading to a more thorough understanding of CWD.

3. Implement Ethical Wildlife Management Practices: One of the most important aspects of treating CWD is the ethical handling of affected species. Wildlife management organizations should prioritize humane culling procedures and seek alternative strategies to reduce the impact on

individual animals while efficiently managing the spread of the disease. Recognizing the importance of ecosystems in preventing disease, ethical practices also include protecting biodiversity and habitat integrity. Building a shared responsibility for the welfare of wildlife and the environment requires public participation in wildlife conservation initiatives and ethical considerations.

4. Encourage Cooperation and Information Sharing: Overcoming disciplinary and geographic barriers, a collaborative approach is necessary to address CWD. Information and best practices should be actively shared by the public, non-profit groups, governments, and scholars. Collaboration platforms have the potential to expedite the advancement of CWD management by enabling the interchange of knowledge, resources, and experience. Collaboration and communication that are transparent will fortify our group's response to this changing problem.

In conclusion, a coordinated and aggressive reaction is required to counter the threat posed by zombie deer illness. Through the implementation of ethical wildlife management methods, promoting public awareness, funding research and monitoring, and encouraging cooperation, stakeholders may work together to mitigate the effects of CWD on animals and protect public health. This call to action acts as a focal point for a group effort to solve the problems caused by zombie deer illness and clear the path for a resilient and sustainable future for communities and animals alike.